KETOGENIC DIET

55 BUDGET-FRIENDLY RECIPES TO LOSE WEIGHT

A Low Carb Cookbook for Beginners

Adele Baker

Dedication

Dedicated to my family:

To my loving husband, who never stopped believing in me, no matter what I said or did

To my little daughter, my inspiration and my soul

Many thanks to my mentor, A.P., for passing this way with me, from the beginning to the end.

Letter to the Reader

The crisp air, pungent with the scent of decaying leaves, envelopes my daughter and I. "More leaves, Mama!" she shrieks with joy. Our favourite activity this year, a pastime of the ages, is to rake enormous piles of leaves so that I can lift her high and toss her into the middle. We spend hours this way, taking joy in each other's presence. I am grateful for the gift of health and life.

Born in Virginia, my family moved to northern Michigan at age 5, to live among sand dunes, ski resorts and hiking trails. My parents' priorities were to enjoy family life and to experience the world. They fostered a love of nature, and we hiked the Blue Ridge mountains, the Alps, and the Carpathians.

When my daughter was 12 months old, I began the trek toward a serious change of lifelong eating habits. My clothes were painfully tight around the waist. It had been a full year since giving birth, and the pregnancy weight I'd accumulated was not going to magically melt away. My adventures began with the ketogenic diet and will continue for the rest of my life. After considering various diets, I acknowledged the ketogenic diet would best fit my lifestyle. Scouring books and consulting the internet for recipes, I came up short.

Today, I have acquired and perfected delicious recipes for every meal, and made them available to fellow keto dieters. My hope is that you, too, will discover the joy of a slimmer, healthier body.

Introduction

The fact that you have picked up this book tells us that you have tried the odd diet or two in the past and did not see the results you had hoped for. It's no surprise that countless people try several diets before they find one that works for them, and sometimes, they give up on the idea altogether.

There's no need to give up!

There is a diet out there that suits you, and suits your lifestyle. The thing that most people struggle with, however, is hunger.

Have you ever been on a diet, but you didn't feel hungry? Have you ever been on a diet and wanted to bite everyone's heads off because you felt so irritable with sugar cravings that you simply couldn't think straight?

Do you want some good news?

We know a diet that doesn't have a horrendous side effect, and still allows you to lose the weight you want, and probably a bit more for good measure.

Yes, seriously, this is no joke.

Have you heard of the ketogenic diet? You might have heard of it referred to as the keto diet for short, and for ease, that's what we will continue to call it. This is basically a low carbohydrate diet, which switches your body's primary source of fuel from carbs to fat. The result? You're burning fat for energy, and because you're eating more fat in your diet to compensate, you're less likely to suffer the same hunger and cravings you would have on a regular low calorie diet.

How Does the Keto Diet Work?

You might be a little confused at this point, wondering how something which sounds so good could actually be true. Well, let's explain a bit more about how it all works, and then you will see the science behind it.

Your body is programed to burn carbs for energy. This means that your body sends fuel, which is a result of burning carbohydrates, to your vital organs. This fuel enables them to work, as well as to give you the power to be able to move and go about your daily business. The keto diet turns off that switch and instead of burning carbs, your body burns fat. This happens by limiting the number of carbs you eat, and your body then naturally switches to the next sensible source of fuel, which is fat.

Ketosis is the process which begins this switch from burning carbs to burning fat. While ketosis is not dangerous if you follow the diet properly, it does have a brief period of side effects. You will need to learn how to minimize the side effects in order to get to the clear air on the other side. We will talk in more detail about managing side effects later in the book. For now, you simply need to know that on this diet you are very unlikely to be hungry or to have cravings, because you are going to be eating more fat, and fat content foods are much more satisfying than low-calorie or low-fat foods.

In a short amount of time, you will be burning fat as your primary source of fuel, which means that you will be making quick and effective headway into stored fat. These are the parts of your body that are squishy and annoying. Before you know it, you will have that beach body!

How is the Keto Diet Different from Other Low Calorie Diets?

It's vitally important to realise that the keto diet is not a quick fix fad diet. It is actually a lifestyle change that you will want to continue for the rest of your life. The keto diet will teach you how to eat 'clean' foods, e.g. foods which have not been affected by pesticides, antibiotics, or anything artificial. Instead, the emphasis is on natural ingredients and organics. You will have improved health from the start.

The keto diet differs from low calorie diets because it is sustainable, and it gives much more choice in terms of what you eat. Many low calorie diets are very restrictive, and if you've ever been on one, you have probably had one or two moments where you rebelled completely, and eventually threw in the towel. This is because your body simply cannot handle that amount of restriction over a long period of time.

Low calorie diets mean that you keep calories in your daily food low, but you are still burning carbs. This doesn't make much headway into stored fat reserves, and any progress is likely to be slow. For this reason, that many people fail.

What Are the Benefits of the Keto Diet?

Let's break it down into simple benefits:
- ✓ Fast, effective weight loss
- ✓ Less hunger or cravings
- ✓ Level metabolism, with no sugar spikes
- ✓ Increased quality of sleep
- ✓ Increased focus and concentration
- ✓ More energy - a lot more!
- ✓ Increased knowledge about your general health and well-being
- ✓ Sustainable life-style
- ✓ Decreased risk of developing type II diabetes

✓ Evidence that the keto diet can help to lower blood pressure

How to Follow the Keto Diet

The keto diet is easy to follow: You simply learn the foods you can eat, the ones you can't, and the ones you can have in moderation. Once you know all of this, and over time it will become second nature, you can easily find countless delicious meals and snacks to enjoy. It's important to make sure you get your daily allowance of protein, as this works hand in hand with the diet to ensure it not only works, but that your health is optimized also.

Currently, the daily allowance of protein stands at 0.8 grams of protein per kilo of body weight, or 0.36 grams per pound. As you lose weight, you will need to adjust your protein intake accordingly.

Ready to Begin?

Over the coming chapters, we're going to give you countless hints and tips on how to follow the keto diet successfully, as well as show you some delicious recipes you can enjoy.

So, without further ado, let's begin your journey to health, well-being, and a slimmer waistline

Chapter 1 The Ketogenic Lifestyle – Budget Friendly Ingredients

When you hear the words 'organic', 'clean foods', and 'grass fed', you might go into a panic thinking that the foods you're going to need to purchase as part of your diet are going to be expensive. If you're on a budget, that's not something you need to hear!

The good news? The keto diet is not going to cost you the earth, as most of the fresh, healthy ingredients can be found for a low price tag from your local grocery store. You will need to ensure that the foods you purchase follow the guidelines in terms of how they have been grown, or how they have been reared, in the case of meat. In a moment, we're going to go through the foods you can and cannot eat on the keto diet, as well as the foods which you can eat in moderation. You'll see from these lists what we're talking about in terms of 'clean foods'. You will need to avoid anything with added nasties, e.g. pesticides, antibiotics, additives, or colorings.

Foods You Can Eat Freely

- ✓ Meats – Anything which has been grass-fed, e.g. beef, goat, venison, lamb
- ✓ Wild-caught fish/seafood – Avoid anything factory farmed
- ✓ Pork products which are pastured
- ✓ Poultry products, such as chicken or turkey, and eggs which are free range and pastured
- ✓ Ghee
- ✓ Butter
- ✓ Saturated fats
- ✓ Monounsaturated fats
- ✓ Grass-fed animal organ meat, e.g. kidney
- ✓ Leafy greens, e.g. spinach, lettuce

- ✓ Cucumber
- ✓ Asparagus
- ✓ Bamboo shoots
- ✓ Celery
- ✓ Dressings, e.g. things like mayonnaise, sauerkraut
- ✓ Spices
- ✓ Herbs
- ✓ Water
- ✓ Black coffee
- ✓ Herbal/Black tea

Foods You Can Enjoy in Moderation

- ✓ Cruciferous vegetables, along the lines of cauliflower, Brussel sprouts etc
- ✓ Tomatoes
- ✓ Peppers
- ✓ Aubergine
- ✓ Certain root vegetables, e.g. leeks, onions, pumpkin, garlic
- ✓ Water chestnuts
- ✓ Beansprouts
- ✓ Strawberries
- ✓ Blackberries
- ✓ Coconut
- ✓ Olives
- ✓ Rhubarb
- ✓ Full fat dairy products
- ✓ Meats which have come from a grain-fed animal
- ✓ Bacon
- ✓ Nuts
- ✓ Sugar-free tomato products, such as ketchup
- ✓ Melon
- ✓ Alcoholic spirits, provided they are unsweetened
- ✓ Dry wines, e.g. red or white

Foods You Cannot Eat on the Keto Diet

✓ Any type of grain product, such as white potatoes, pizzas, bulgur wheat, oats, corn, pizzas, pasta, etc
✓ Sugary sauces
✓ Breadcrumbs
✓ Meat which has been factory farmed
✓ High mercury content fish
✓ Battery farmed poultry
✓ Battery farmed eggs
✓ Chocolate
✓ Sweets
✓ Ice cream
✓ Puddings
✓ Cakes
✓ Sugary soft drinks, including diet versions or low sugar
✓ Processed food of any type
✓ Artificial sweeteners
✓ Low-fat milk or skimmed milk
✓ Half fat oils or fats
✓ Exotic fruits, e.g. banana, pineapple, kiwi, mango
✓ Fruit juices
✓ Dried fruits
✓ Alcoholic drinks which are high in sugar content

It's a good idea to print off these pages and keep them in your bag, purse, or wallet, so that when you're out shopping in the first few weeks of starting the keto diet, you can refer to them. This means you won't make any mistakes or waste money on items you shouldn't be eating.You might be staring in shock at the list of foods you can't eat. Let's call them our 'red danger' foods and drinks. But there is no diet on this earth that will let you eat whatever you want and keep its promise of weight loss at the end of it. You need to bear in mind that the keto diet is about changing your lifestyle for good, e.g. learning towards health and wellbeing, and not simply trying a diet for a few months, until you reach the desired number on your scales, and then going back to your old ways. Chocolates, sweets, and pizzas are not healthy, so you shouldn't be eating them – it's that simple!

Later in this book we are going to go over a few recipes you can try as part of your keto diet. You will see that there are more than enough delicious and tasty foods you can eat, enough to keep your mind off those you might think you'll miss. If it helps, try to imagine those red-light foods as being bad, nasty, dirty, even toxic. If you can put a label on them and create an unsavoury image when you think of them, your brain will bring that picture into your head. You will no longer want those foods, because they evoke a disgusting image. The ketogenic diet is about training your mind as well as your body.

General Guidelines to Bear in Mind

✓ All food you consume on the keto diet needs to be clean, and this means nothing added in during the growing or manufacturing process. Meat needs to be grass fed, eggs need to have come from a happy hen, e.g. one which was able to run free, and wasn't caged. The same goes for vegetables and fruit. They need to have been grown in the most natural way possible, without chemical enhancements.

✓ Every recipe you make needs to have no more than 10 grams of net carbs per serving. You need to pay attention to **net carbs** and not total carbs, as this is what we use to measure on this particular diet.

✓ Every food you eat needs to be low carbohydrate content, so you are helping your body stay in that state of ketosis, burning fat instead of carbs for energy.

✓ You should make sure you get your daily recommended amount of protein in your diet every single day, without fail.

✓ Mix up the types of foods you eat, to avoid boredom, and also to keep a variation of vitamins and minerals in your diet.

✓ Drink plenty of water, not only to stay hydrated, but to keep your digestive system happy and healthy.

Keto Shopping on a Budget

The key to finding fresh, organic, clean foods while on a budget is to shop around. Fresh fruit and vegetable markets are the best places to go; supermarkets do have regular deliveries, but their produce is not as fresh as those which are sold from farmer's markets. This is just a fact, and this is what keeps smaller concerns in business. You could argue that you're doing your bit for the local economy by shopping at markets, rather than at grocery stores.

Don't overbuy, because organic food doesn't last as long as fruit and vegetables which have been treated with chemicals. This is a doubled-edged sword, because the fact that they are untreated means they are fresher and better for you. But because they don't last as long, you could argue that they cost you more if they rot before you use them. Simply buy what you need and use it all up. It's also a good idea to plan meals at the beginning of the week.

The main advantages of meal plans are:

✓ You cut down on the chances of impulse buying.
✓ You save time because you know exactly what you're going to make for dinner.
✓ You can do some preparation the night before, e.g. slicing and refrigerating ingredients.
✓ You are less likely to make unhealthy choices simply because you don't know what to eat that evening.
✓ You are also less likely to make unhealthy choices because you won't be walking around the supermarket hungry.

✓ If you have had a long day at work, knowing what you are going to make when you get home is a much less stressful situation.
✓ You can buy your ingredients slightly ahead of time and you know you're not going to waste anything, which saves cash, and helps the environment.

Now you know what you can and can't eat, and you know how to shop sensibly, we'll move onto a few more tips to help you get into the keto diet quicker and easier.

Chapter 2 Cutlery & Gadgets

The best ketogenic kitchen needs some gadgets and household items to make life easier. The fact that you're going to be cooking a majority of your meals and snacks from scratch means that you need the best accessories to help you do that!

There are certain key pieces of equipment that you need, as well as a few optional things which will make life easier. As a general rule, these are the items you should have on hand:

✓ **Food processor** – This is a must have for every keto kitchen! Whether you're chopping, blending, or doing something else entirely, a food processor is going to make life easier. You don't need the most up-to-date type of machine, but you do need something which is going to stand up to a lot of use. As a bonus, smoothies are also easy to do in a food processor.
✓ **A freestanding mixer** – A mixer is another must have, and we're talking about the retro types here, with Kitchenaid having a wide variety to offer. This is for mixing and combining, as well as blending. This type of machine is ideal for dessert recipes, and you'll be wanting some of those.
✓ **High quality knives** – You're going to do a lot of chopping and cutting, and if you have blunt, poor quality

knives, the whole process is going to be frustrating at best. It's worth spending a little extra cash here, because quality knives are a necessity.

✓ **An immersion blender** – Soups are a staple of the keto diet, and a hand-held immersion blender will help you mix up delicious meals in no time. To try to make a keto soup without this piece of equipment is difficult, messy and time consuming.

✓ **Vegetable slicer** – Unless you want to spend hours doing this manually, a vegetable slicer will be a big timesaver.

✓ **A set of cutting boards** – Again, go for quality here and make sure you get a set of boards, because you can then avoid the worries about cross contamination and improper cleaning. Again, you're going to be chopping a lot of things, including fruits, vegetables, herbs, and meat, so you need quality boards to carry out your work.

✓ **Quality kitchen shears** – For deboning chicken, slicing up bacon, chopping vegetables, shears are a staple of the keto kitchen.

✓ **Mini whisks** – Keto cooks will tell you that eggs are a prominent ingredient in many recipes. You'll be needing to whisk a lot, so having a small set of easy-to-grab and easy-to-use whisks is a good idea. They will help achieve that light and fluffy consistency.

✓ **Small prep bowls** – If you have a busy life, e.g. you want to do your lunches for work the night before, or you're pushed for time, you can do some prep for your meals when you're not so busy. Having small prep bowls will help you keep everything organised.

✓ **Measuring spoons** – Definite necessities! All diets place importance on correct measurements. The proper piece of equipment will certainly help you in that regard.

✓ **Avocado slicer** –Avocados are prevalent in the keto diet, and you don't have to be a brain surgeon to know that peeling, de-stoning, and slicing an avocado isn't easy without some kind of aid.

✓ **Measuring cups** – Just like the measuring spoons, measuring cups are crucial, to ensure that you get all of those measurements right.

✓ **Food scales** – You can find mini versions of this piece of equipment, but it's worth spending a little cash here. The best scales will give you information on nutritional content as well as portion size information, and this is helpful for those with a busy life.

✓ **Psyllium husk powder** – This is not a piece of equipment per se, but it is something that every keto kitchen needs. This will revolutionize your keto cooking, and is something you need to keep in your cupboards. Psyllium husk powder can be used to give your recipes the feel of anything which would normally have wheat in it, because you can't have the wheat. It can also be used as a thickener or in sweet recipes. A super ingredient!

These are a few ideas of things which your new keto kitchen should have, and these will help you create delicious recipes that we're going to go discuss later.

Chapter 3 Tips & Tricks for Beginners

When you start something new, it's totally normal to feel a little overwhelmed by the dos, don'ts, hints, tips, and everything else thrown in for good measure. When starting the keto diet, the best advice is to do plenty of reading up on it first, then determine your understanding of things. From there you can work through the first phases, without being confused by stories coming from here, there, and everywhere.

It's important to give yourself time and understanding: this is a huge deal. It is a big change of lifestyle, so be sure to take it slowly and follow advice from reputable sources.

When you start the keto diet, you will be like a sponge – ready to soak up all the hints and tips you can find! Of course, the first part of the diet is the hardest, because this is when the diet is most restrictive, and this is also when your body is starting its re-programing, changing its primary fuel source from carbs to fats. When you start anything new, be it a new job, or driving a new car, you need to give yourself a little time to adjust, and some would call this the transitional period. The keto diet is no different; when you push your body into ketosis, there is a period of slight shock for your body, and this is when you might experience a few side effects.

The Side Effects of The Keto Diet

All of the side effects you may experience in the first phase of the keto diet are reversible to a degree, and all of them should be short-lived. We stress the point that if you experience any effects which are particularly unpleasant, prolonged, or anything you're worried about, seek medical advice without delay. If you have any health issues, it's always important to speak to your doctor before you begin the diet.

Pep talk over, here are the main side effects which are common during the first month of the keto diet.

✓ **Needing to use the bathroom, a lot**

This is the most common side effect of them all, and there is a scientific reason behind it! It might be annoying, and you might need to be within close proximity to a toilet wherever you go, but it's actually a good thing! When you first go into ketosis, your body kicks out a lot of excess fluid, and your kidneys also release extra stored fluids too. All of this means you're going to need the toilet more than normal, but over time this should ease off.

How to minimize it? You can't really minimize it, but you can do something help avoid dehydration. Keep drinking water – yes, that is going to send you back to the bathroom, but you need to keep your fluids up. It's also a good idea to salt your food, literally on everything you can, because this will replace the sodium minerals you're losing.

✓ **Feeling a little dizzy**

Again, this is the transition your body is going through, which is going to make your whole system feel a little out of whack for a few weeks. This could also be down to the sodium loss, through peeing more often, so again, salt your food and make sure you drink plenty of water to stay hydrated. You might also feel a little tired or lacking in energy, but the good news is that when the diet's positive effects kick in, you're going to be bursting with energy!

Eating potassium rich foods, such as avocados, should help with the dizziness and lethargy.

✓ **Headaches**

If you get severe headaches, or you find these are extremely often, you should seek advice. But generally speaking, a slight increase in headaches is common during the first month of the keto diet.

There are a few reasons into why this could be the case. It could be due to the loss of sodium, or it could be due to dehydration. By now, you know the answer to this – drink plenty of water and salt your food! Potassium will help you here, too.

✓ **Constipation issues**

You might find that you become constipated during the first phase, but this is due to the change in your eating habits, and will happen with any dietary change you make in your life. Drinking plenty of water can help you out with constipation, as well as salt intake, but a magnesium supplement might be an option also.

✓ **Muscle cramps**

This is probably the most common complaint by people who begin the diet, but it should ease off quite quickly. This is a mineral loss issue, again due to excessive urination. Drink plenty of water, salt your food (yes, again!), and if you are struggling, think about taking a magnesium citrate supplement to help you along.

✓ **Sleep disruption issues**

This is something that will change as your body becomes used to the diet. You're making big changes to the way your body is used to running its daily business, and everything will be a little haywire at first. Your sleep pattern is probably going to be one of the first things to go a little out of whack, and relaxation is the key to overcoming sleep disruption.

Enjoy a warm drink before bed, relax as much as you can, turn off your phone, chill out, get comfortable, read a book, do whatever it takes to help yourself relax. It's important not to get too stressed about this issue, because it certainly will ease as time moves on.

✓ **Sugar cravings – but only at first!**

You might be thinking 'What?! You said I wouldn't crave sugar!' but in the first period you might, a little. This is again because your body is wondering what on earth is going on, but once your body settles down, those cravings will, too. The only way to conquer this is to put mind over matter, and remember why you're doing this. You can get through this initial period!

The power to get through the first part of the diet, when the side effects might be a little more prevalent, it something that you need to find within. Yes, we've mentioned the ways to minimize the side effects, mainly drinking water and salting food, but a lot of it is also mind over matter. You have to have faith in the process, you need to trust that your body is just doing what it needs to do in order to adjust and refocus its attention. It will begin to burn that fat for energy just as you're instructing it to do by forcing it into ketosis.

It's also important to remember that ketosis is not dangerous, provided you follow the diet as it is meant to be followed.

In addition to the advice we've given regarding side effects, the following tips will help you kick start your keto diet adventure.

✓ **Keep your water levels up** – We have talked about this in terms of side effects, but in terms of helping the keto diet actually work, hydration is vital. It's easy to get so busy during your day that you forget to keep drinking. It's important to remember that you need to think about what you're drinking, as much as how often. Avoid sugary drinks, even if they say they are diet or low fat drinks, and stick to pure water as much as possible.

✓ **Keep your salt levels up** – Again, we mentioned this earlier, but we also need to highlight how salt helps the diet. You might think that this advice contradicts what we are told in society, i.e. don't eat too much salt, but on the keto diet you need to eat salt! When you are on a higher carb diet, e.g. a low-calorie diet, you have higher insulin levels, which means that your kidneys keep sodium (salt) in your body. When you are on a low carb diet, such as the keto diet, you have naturally lower insulin levels, so your kidneys kick out the sodium rather than holding it in, and therefore you need to replenish this to maintain good health. Pink Himalayan salt is a good addition to your diet, as this has many other advantages aside from replenishing your sodium levels.

✓ **Exercise is key** – No diet works alone without exercise. Exercise has many advantages overall, and it is crucial for your health and well-being. On the keto diet, exercise will help boost your glut-4 receptor in the liver, which helps extract sugar from the main bloodstream, to be stored in the liver and muscles instead. This is a boost in ketosis, so exercise is a must.

✓ **Get your protein intake, but don't go overboard** – Protein is important, but if you eat too much, the body will turn the amino acid in the protein into glucose. This will disrupt the ketogenic process. Your aim should be 0.8 grams per kilogram of your body weight. For example: A 125 pound woman (56.7 kilograms) should eat 56.7*0.8=46 grams of protein per day.

✓ **Stay de-stressed as much as possible** –We live busy lives, and sometimes stress is unavoidable, but levels which are too high become unsafe, and will wreak havoc with your ketosis. This is because when you are stressed, your stress hormones go through the roof, and which, in turn, increases your blood sugar. When this happens for a prolonged period of time, not only is this dangerous, but it won't help your dieting at all because high blood pressure and lower levels of ketones won't help ketosis either.

✓ **Look after yourself** – The keto diet is about a lifestyle change, and a lifestyle change is about the whole package, including how you eat, how you exercise, how you keep your stress down, and how you look after yourself in terms of finding time for you, and getting enough sleep. Don't put yourself last. It's not selfish to look after yourself!

These are just a few hints and tips which will help you kick-start your keto adventure. In the next chapter, we are going to talk about the common mistakes that people make on the keto diet, and how to avoid them.

Chapter 4 Common Mistakes & How to Avoid Them

It's normal to make a few mistakes when you start a new endeavour, whether you've read all the literature out there or not! Don't beat yourself up if you stumble a little, but it's important to recognise when you're making mistakes. You will probably notice this at first because you're not losing the weight you thought, or perhaps you are experiencing more in the way of side effects.

Again, we need to reiterate one very important point – if you are at all worried about side effects, or anything you are experiencing, talk to your doctor immediately. Also, remember to talk with your doctor about the diet before starting, if you have any pre-existing conditions.

There are common mistakes that people tend to make when they start the keto diet, so let us be your guide to avoiding them!

Common mistake 1 – Not eating enough protein

We have mentioned this one before – you need to get your protein amount per kilogram of your body weight, and you need to adjust this as you lose weight. Protein is vital for your health, not only on this diet, but on any diet, and if you are working out, this is even more important!

Common mistake 2 – Eating too much protein

On the other hand, too much protein is not good either! Your body is going to convert the protein into glucose (sugar) and that will affect the ketosis state that your body needs to be in. Stick to the recommended amount, which is .8 grams per kilogram of body weight, and you'll be fine.

Common mistake 3 – Not exercising

No diet works without exercise, and exercise is good for your health. Grab a friend and go for a run, join an exercise class, or join the gym. You could even play a team sport-- anything that gets your blood pumping. All of this will help your muscles tone as you lose weight, too.

Common mistake 4 – Not mixing up your meals enough

You need a range of options, otherwise you're just going to get bored and the whole dieting process will become a chore. Remember that this is a lifestyle change, and for that reason you need variety.

Common mistake 5 – Viewing the keto diet as a fad choice

We have said this so many times so far – the keto diet is a lifestyle change! You are committing to a life of healthier choices, clean foods, and working out, because this is all better for your health and well-being. If you're looking for a quick fix, the keto diet isn't for you!

Common mistake 6 – Becoming super obsessed with the scales

Step away from those scales! You should only weigh yourself once a week, and if you are obsessed with weighing yourself every morning, you need to stop. Your weight naturally fluctuates on a daily basis, especially if you are a woman, so once a week should be your aim and your measurement.

Common mistake 7 – Getting confused over total carbs and net carbs

We'll simplify this right down – when measuring it all out on the keto diet, you're paying attention to net carbs only.

Common mistake 8 – Not getting enough fats, or the wrong kinds

If you're not eating enough fats, especially the right kinds (saturated) then you are going to push your body back into the carb burning side, and you're not going to be burning fat. This is going to sabotage all your efforts and cause total chaos with your metabolism.

Common mistake 9 – Comparing yourself with others

If anything is going to sabotage your efforts, it's your own mind. Do not compare yourself to anyone, and certainly don't compare your progress to anyone else's. This is a personal issue, and you need to concentrate on your own efforts.

Common mistake 10 – Not getting enough salt

Around 2 teaspoons of salt per day should be consumed on the keto diet. Unlike a low-calorie diet, you won't be overloaded with salt, you will be deficient in it. Salt your food and this problem will be overcome.

There you have it, ten common mistakes and how to avoid them. Of course, there are probably a few more, which are respective to you, but the main advice we can give is to follow the guidelines as they are set out, and to give yourself an area of choice in terms of your food. You need to mix it up, you need to give yourself variation, and provided your meals are keto friendly, i.e. low carb, high fat, you're getting enough protein (but not too much), and you're getting enough salt, you're good to go!

Speaking of good to go, let's move on to give you some delicious and easy to use recipes, to help you get started on this epic journey toward health and well-being!

Chapter 5 5-10 Minute Recipes

In this chapter, we will give you ten delicious recipes to try. They only take around 5-10 minutes to prepare – ideal for those who are in a rush! These recipes are ideal for breakfast, snacks, or for salad/soup meal options.

Low Carb Caramel

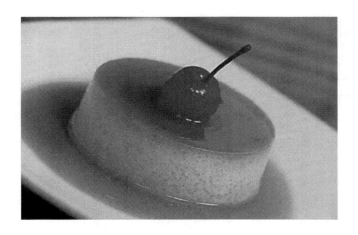

| Category – Snacks | Cooking time – 5 min |
| Servings - 4 | Preparation time - 5 min |

Ingredients

4 tablespoons unsalted butter

4 tablespoons heavy cream

1 teaspoon erythritol

Salt, 1 pinch

Preparation Method

✓ Melt the butter until it turns golden.

✓ Add the heavy cream and stir, keeping the pan on a lower heat.

✓ Mix in the erythritol until it dissolves completely.

✓ Add the salt to the pan.

✓ The mixture is finished once it is thick.

Nutritional information

✓ Fat per serving – 17 grams

✓ Net carbs per serving – 1/2 gram

✓ Protein per serving – 0 grams

✓ Calories per serving – 163 calories

Blueberry Ricotta Pancakes

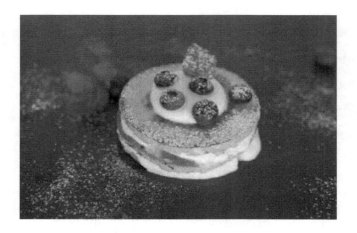

| Category – Breakfast | Cooking time – 5 min |
| Servings - 5 | Preparation time - 5 min |

Ingredients

3 eggs

¾ cup ricotta

1/2 teaspoon vanilla extract

1/4 cup unsweetened almond milk

1 cup almond flour

1/2 cup golden flaxseed meal

1/4 teaspoon salt

1 teaspoon baking powder

1/4 teaspoon stevia powder

1/4 cup blueberries

Preparation Method

✓ Preheat your skillet to medium.

✓ Combine the eggs, ricotta, vanilla extract and almond milk.

✓ In a separate bowl, mix together the almond flour, flaxseed meal, salt, baking powder and stevia.

✓ Slowly, add the flour mixture to the blended ingredients. Blend until smooth.

✓ Halve the blueberries.

✓ Stir half the blueberries into the batter.

✓ Melt the butter in the skillet.

✓ Scoop ¼ cup of the mixture into the pan for each pancake, and when browned on the first side, flip.

✓ Serve and sprinkle berries on top.

Nutritional information

✓ Fat per serving – 22.6 grams

✓ Net carbs per serving – 5.9 grams

✓ Protein per serving – 13.4 grams

✓ Calories per serving – 296.6 calories

Pesto Chicken Salad

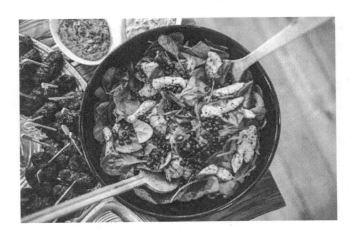

| Category – Salads | Cooking time – 2 min |
| Servings - 1 | Preparation time - 5 min |

Ingredients

1 pound chicken, cooked and cubed

6 slices of bacon, cooked and crumbled into small pieces

1 cubed avocado

10 halved cherry tomatoes

1/4 cup mayonnaise

2 tablespoon garlic pesto

lettuce leaves

Preparation Method

- ✓ In a large bowl, combine the chicken, bacon, avocado, tomatoes, mayonnaise and pesto.

- ✓ Spoon the mixture on top of lettuce leaves and serve.

Nutritional information

- ✓ Fat per serving – 27 grams

- ✓ Net carbs per serving – 3 grams

- ✓ Protein per serving – 27 grams

- ✓ Calories per serving – 375 calories

Cobb Salad

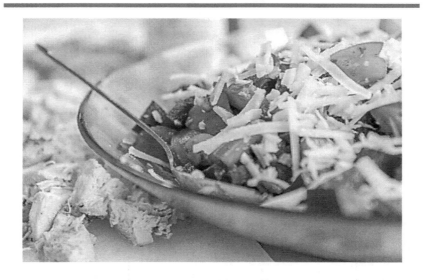

| Category – Salads | Cooking time – 2 min |
| Servings - 1 | Preparation time - 5 min |

Ingredients

1 cup spinach

1 hard-boiled egg

2 cooked bacon strips

2 ounces chicken breast, cooked

½ Campari tomato

¼ avocado

½ teaspoon white vinegar

1 tablespoon olive oil

Preparation Method

✓ Slice up the chicken and bacon.

✓ Chop the other ingredients into small pieces.

✓ Combine everything together in a large mixing bowl with the oil and vinegar.

✓ Toss and serve.

Nutritional information

✓ Fat per serving – 48 grams

✓ Net carbs per serving – 3 grams

✓ Protein per serving – 43 grams

✓ Calories per serving – 600 calories

Grilled Halloumi Salad

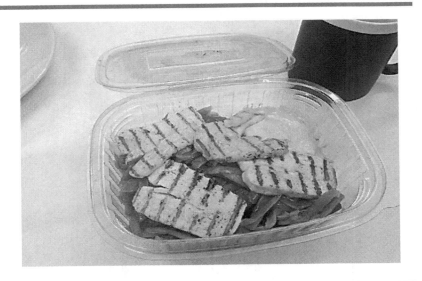

Category – Salads Servings - 4	Cooking time – 5 min Preparation time - 5 min

Ingredients

3 ounces Halloumi cheese

1 cucumber

5 cherry tomatoes

One handful baby arugula

5 ounces chopped walnuts

Olive oil

Balsamic vinegar

Salt

Preparation Method

✓ Cut the halloumi into thick slices.

✓ The cheese should be grilled for around 4 minutes on each side, until lines appear.

✓ Prepare the salad ingredients in a bowl.

✓ Place the grilled halloumi over the salad.

✓ Dress the dish with olive oil, balsamic vinegar, and salt.

Nutritional information

✓ Fat per serving – 10.4 grams

✓ Net carbs per serving – 7.3 grams

✓ Protein per serving – 3 grams

✓ Calories per serving – 134 calories

Watermelon Cream Soup

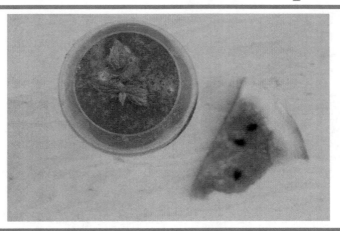

Category – Soups	Cooking time – 5 min
Servings - 1	Preparation time - 5 min

Ingredients

¾ cup watermelon, deseeded, cut into chunks

¼ cup raspberries

2 tablespoons sour cream

1 tablespoon sugar-free vanilla bean sweetener

juice of ¼ lemon

¼ teaspoon fresh mint, chopped

½ cup whipped cream

Preparation Method

✓ Combine all the ingredients in a blender; using the pulse function, blend until smooth.

✓ Pour the mixture into a bowl.

✓ Serve and enjoy!

Nutritional information

✓ Fat per serving – 17 grams

✓ Net carbs per serving – 8 grams

✓ Protein per serving – 2 grams

✓ Calories per serving – 192 calories

Strawberry Pistachio Creamsicles

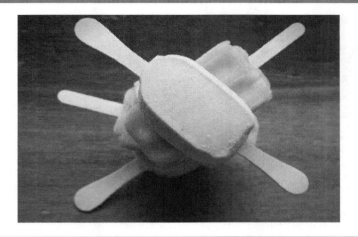

Category – Snacks	Cooking time – 2 min
Servings - 4	Preparation time - 2 min

Ingredients

8 ounces strawberries

2 ounces salted pistachios

½ cup heavy cream

½ cup almond milk

2 teaspoons stevia

Preparation Method

✓ Combine the strawberries, stevia, heavy cream, and almond milk in a blender.

✓ Add the pistachios and stir well.

✓ Pour the mixture into popsicle molds.

✓ Freeze for around 2 hours.

Nutritional information

✓ Fat per serving – 12.5 grams

✓ Net carbs per serving – 5.6 grams

✓ Protein per serving – 4 grams

✓ Calories per serving – 158 calories

Guacamole

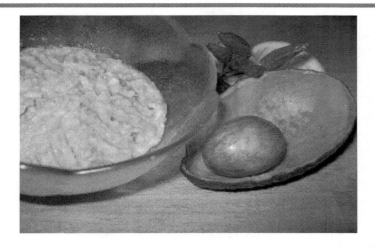

Category – Snacks	Cooking time – 5 min
Servings – 1.5	Preparation time - 10 min

Ingredients

2 avocados

¼ cup of diced onions

6 cherry tomatoes

2 cloves garlic

1 tablespoon olive oil

Juice of half a lime

¼ teaspoon salt

1/8 teaspoon black pepper

1/8 teaspoon crushed red pepper

Fresh parsley

Fresh cilantro

Preparation Method

- ✓ Mash the avocado.
- ✓ Add the onion and tomatoes to the mixture (small pieces).
- ✓ Add the chopped garlic and stir well.
- ✓ Add the spices and stir well.
- ✓ Add the parsley and cilantro, and stir well.
- ✓ Mix in the lime juice and stir well.

Nutritional information

- ✓ Fat per serving – 7 grams
- ✓ Net carbs per serving – 1 gram
- ✓ Protein per serving – 1 gram
- ✓ Calories per serving – 77 calories

Tropical Smoothie

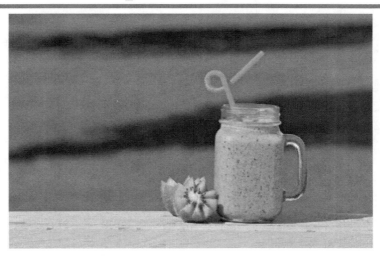

Category – Brackrast/Snacks	Cooking time – 2 min
Servings – 1	Preparation time - 3 min

Ingredients

7 ice cubes

¾ cup coconut milk

¼ cup sour cream

2 tablespoons golden flaxseed meal

1 tablespoons MCT oil

20 drops liquid stevia

½ teaspoons mango extract

¼ teaspoon blueberry extract

¼ teaspoon banana extract

Preparation Method

✓ Blend all the ingredients together on a pulse action.

✓ Blend the mixture on high for one minute, until a thick consistency occurs.

✓ Pour and serve!

Nutritional information

✓ Fat per serving – 31 grams

✓ Net carbs per serving – 3 grams

✓ Protein per serving – 5 grams

✓ Calories per serving – 352 calories

Quick Boiled Eggs

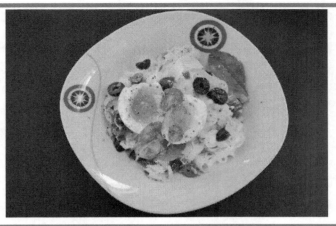

Category – Brackrast/Snacks	Cooking time – 2 min
Servings – 1	Preparation time - 3 min

Ingredients

2 eggs

Salt, Pepper

1 teaspoon mayonnaise

2 ham deli slices

Cilantro, a handful

Preparation Method

✓ Boil the eggs to preference.

✓ Season with salt and pepper.

✓ Cut the eggs into halves.

✓ Arrange over the cilantro.

✓ Serve with mayonnaise.

Nutritional information

✓ Fat per serving – 7 grams

✓ Net carbs per serving – 5 grams

✓ Protein per serving – 8 grams

✓ Calories per serving – 135 calories

Chocolate Mousse

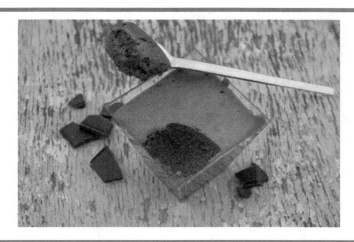

Category – Snacks	Cooking time – 2 min
Servings – 3	Preparation time - 10 min

Ingredients

1 teaspoon cocoa powder, unsweetened,

3-4 tablespoons heavy cream

1 drop vanilla extract

Preparation Method

✓ Mix together the cocoa powder, heavy cream, and
   vanilla extract

✓ Whip until a thick consistency forms

✓ Enjoy!

Nutritional information

- ✓ Fat per serving – 37 grams
- ✓ Net carbs per serving – 1.5 grams
- ✓ Protein per serving – 2 grams
- ✓ Calories per serving – 335 calories

Crispy Cheddar Cheese Crisps

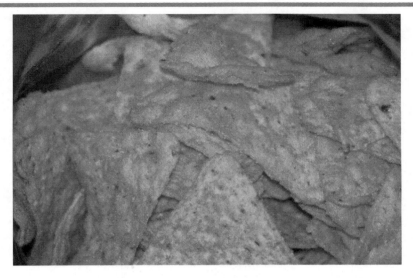

| Category – Snacks | Cooking time – 5 min |
| Servings – 1 | Preparation time - 2 min |

Ingredients

Cheddar cheese, 4 cups

1/2 teaspoon Sea salt

1/2 teaspoon onion powder

1/2 teaspoon garlic powder

¼ teaspoon cumin

¼ teaspoon paprika

¼ teaspoon chili powder

Preparation Method

✓ Preheat the oven to 400°F.

✓ Line a baking tray with parchment.

✓ Combine the cheese and spices.

✓ Spread the mixture out onto the baking tray and form triangles.

✓ Bake for 20 minutes.

✓ Allow to cool

Nutritional information

✓ Fat per serving – 6 grams

✓ Net carbs per serving – 0 grams

✓ Protein per serving – 7 grams

✓ Calories per serving – 90 calories

Anti-Pasto Salad and Easy Italian Dressing

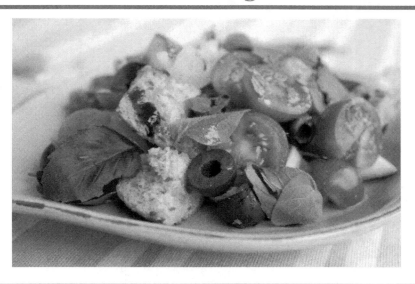

Category – Salads Servings – 2	Cooking time – 2 min Preparation time - 5 min

Ingredients

1 large head Romaine lettuce, chopped

4 ounces prosciutto, cut into strips

4 ounces pepperoni, cut into cubes

½ cup artichoke hearts, sliced

½ cup olives

½ cup sweet peppers, roasted

Italian dressing

Preparation Method

✓ Combine all the ingredients together in a bowl.

✓ Add the Italian dressing to taste.

✓ Mix together well.

✓ Serve!

Nutritional information

✓ Fat per serving – 11 grams

✓ Net carbs per serving – 7 grams

✓ Protein per serving – 19 grams

✓ Calories per serving – 200 calories

Chapter 6 10 to 30 Minute Recipes

Hopefully you'll have given the first ten recipes a try, or at least a few of them, and from there you will have seen just how easy it is to make delicious Keto recipes! Let's take it up a notch now and check out ten recipes which are within the 10 to 30-minute bracket.

Steak and Eggs

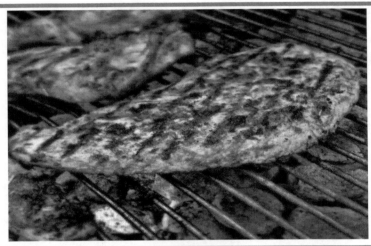

| Category – Lunch/Dinner | Cooking time – 10 min |
| Servings – 1 | Preparation time - 5 min |

Ingredients

1 tablespoon butter

3 eggs

4 ounces lean steak

¼ avocado

Salt

Pepper

Preparation Method

✓ Melt the butter in a hot pan.

✓ Fry the eggs and season.

✓ Cook the steak to your liking.

✓ Once the steak is cooked, season and slice into strips.

✓ Slice the avocado and serve

Nutritional information

✓ Fat per serving – 36 grams

✓ Net carbs per serving – 3 grams

✓ Protein per serving – 44 grams

✓ Calories per serving – 510 calories

Mini Pumpkin Spice Muffins

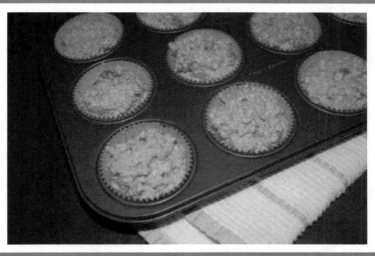

Category – Breakfast/Snack	Cooking time – 15 min
Servings – 16	Preparation time - 15 min

Ingredients

¾ cup canned pumpkin

¼ cup sunflower seed butter

1 egg

½ cup erythritol

¼ cup coconut flour

2 tablespoons flaxseed meal

1 teaspoon ground cinnamon

½ teaspoon ground nutmeg

½ teaspoon baking soda

½ teaspoon salt

Preparation Method

- ✓ Preheat your oven to 350°F.
- ✓ Mix the pumpkin, sunflower seed butter and egg together.
- ✓ Add the dry ingredients and stir together.
- ✓ Prepare a muffin pan.
- ✓ Pour the mixture into the muffin pan.
- ✓ Bake for 15 minutes.
- ✓ Cool and serve!

Nutritional information

- ✓ Fat per serving – 2.9 grams
- ✓ Net carbs per serving – 2.64 grams
- ✓ Protein per serving – 1.8 grams
- ✓ Calories per serving – 42 calories

Coconut Pancakes

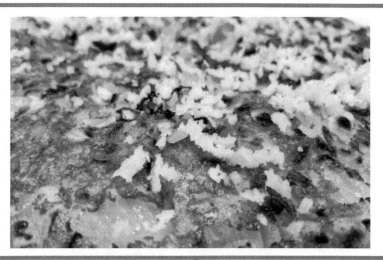

Category – Breakfast/Lunch	Cooking time – 10 min
Servings – 2	Preparation time - 15 min

Ingredients

2 eggs

2 ounces cream cheese

1 tablespoons almond flour

1 teaspoon cinnamon

½ tablespoons erythritol

Salt, just a pinch

¼ cup shredded coconut, unsweetened

2-4 tablespoons maple syrup

Preparation Method

- ✓ Whisk the eggs together.
- ✓ Add the cream cheese and combine well.
- ✓ Add the almond flour, cinnamon, salt, and erythritol, and mix again.
- ✓ Heat a pan on medium and melt half the butter.
- ✓ Scoop ¼ cup of the mixture per pancake onto the skillet.
- ✓ Cook the mixture – it is done when the edges are a little brown on one side; flip over and repeat.
- ✓ Repeat the process with the rest of the mixture.
- ✓ Serve with maple syrup and shredded coconut sprinkled on top.

Nutritional information

- ✓ Fat per serving – 51 grams
- ✓ Net carbs per serving – 3.5 grams
- ✓ Protein per serving – 19 grams
- ✓ Calories per serving – 575 calories

Shakshuka

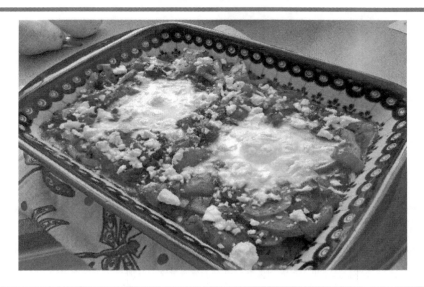

Category – Dinner Servings – 1	Cooking time – 10 min Preparation time - 10 min

Ingredients

1 cup marinara sauce

1 chili pepper

4 eggs

1 ounces feta cheese

1/8 teaspoon cumin

Salt

Pepper

Fresh basil

Preparation Method

- ✓ Preheat your oven to 400°F.
- ✓ Warm a skillet on medium.
- ✓ Cook the marinara sauce and the chopped chili pepper for 5 minutes.
- ✓ Crack the eggs over the skillet pan mixture.
- ✓ Sprinkle the feta cheese over the top.
- ✓ Season with the spices.
- ✓ Bake in the oven for 10 minutes.
- ✓ Serve with chopped fresh basil.

Nutritional information

- ✓ Fat per serving – 34 grams
- ✓ Net carbs per serving – 4 grams
- ✓ Protein per serving – 35 grams
- ✓ Calories per serving – 490 calories

Breakfast Tacos

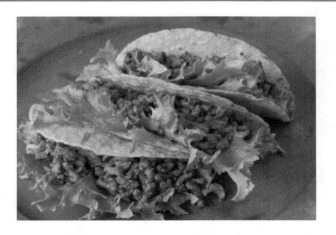

Category – Breakfast Servings – 3	Cooking time – 20 min Preparation time - 10 min

Ingredients

1 cup mozzarella cheese

6 eggs

2 tablespoons butter

3 strips bacon

½ avocado

1 ounces shredded cheddar cheese

Salt

Pepper

Preparation Method

✓ Fry the bacon until crispy, usually around 20 minutes

✓ On a medium heat, warm up 1/3 cup of mozzarella

✓ For the taco shell, fry the cheese until it has browned on the edges, and make sure it doesn't stick by using a spatula to move it occasionally.

✓ Lift up the cheese shell and lay it over a wooden spoon resting on a large pot –Repeat this process until the mixture has been used up.

✓ Cook your eggs and stir; season with salt and pepper.

✓ Add some of the egg mixture to each of your tacos.

✓ Serve with a slice of avocado.

✓ Sprinkle the bacon and shredded cheese over the taco.

Nutritional information

✓ Fat per serving – 36.2 grams

✓ Net carbs per serving – 3 grams

✓ Protein per serving – 25.7 grams

✓ Calories per serving – 443 calories

Tangy Bacon & Egg Salad

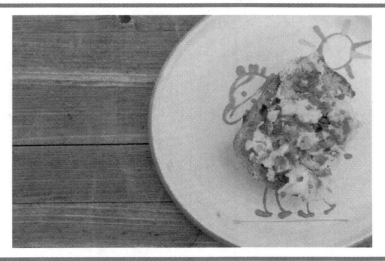

Category – Breakfast/Lunch	Cooking time – 15 min
Servings – 6	Preparation time - 5 min

Ingredients

5 hard-boiled eggs

¼ cup mayonnaise

3 slices bacon

2 tablespoons bacon fat

¼ red onion

2 teaspoons Dijon mustard

¼ teaspoon cayenne pepper

¼ teaspoon black pepper

Preparation Method

- ✓ Slice up the bacon and cook in a pan on a medium heat until crispy.
- ✓ Slice up the red onion.
- ✓ Remove the bacon from the pan and keep the dripping in the pan.
- ✓ Add the bacon dripping to the hard-boiled eggs.
- ✓ Add the red onion, mayonnaise and Dijon mustard to the eggs.
- ✓ Mash the eggs to your liking.
- ✓ Add the cayenne and black pepper, mix together.
- ✓ Add the bacon and fold in gently.
- ✓ Serve

Nutritional information

- ✓ Fat per serving – 30.9 grams
- ✓ Net carbs per serving – 2.1 grams
- ✓ Protein per serving – 15.5 grams
- ✓ Calories per serving – 344 calories

Simple Bacon and Eggs

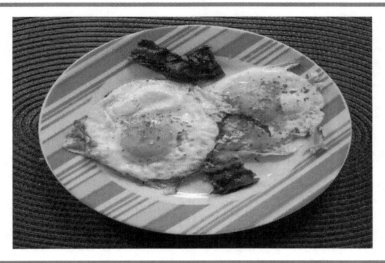

Category – Breakfast/Lunch Servings – 2	Cooking time – 10 min Preparation time - 5 min

Ingredients

3 eggs

1/3 cup heavy cream

1 tablespoon butter

4 slices bacon

Salt

Ground black pepper

Preparation Method

✓ Preheat the oven to 300°F.

✓ Bake the bacon until crispy.

✓ Whisk the eggs together with the cream.

✓ Melt the butter over a medium-low heat.

✓ Add the egg to the pan.

✓ Stir the gently in a figure '8' pattern.

✓ Add the salt and pepper.

✓ Serve with the bacon.

Nutritional information

✓ Fat per serving – 35 grams

✓ Net carbs per serving – 2 grams

✓ Protein per serving – 25 grams

✓ Calories per serving – 444 calories

Savoury Sage and Cheddar Waffles

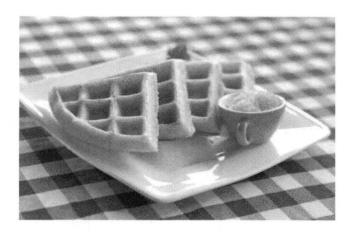

Category – Lunch/Snack Servings – 12	Cooking time – 10 min Preparation time - 20 min

Ingredients

1 1/3 cup coconut flour

3 teaspoons baking powder

1 teaspoon dried ground sage

½ teaspoon salt

¼ teaspoon garlic powder

2 cups coconut milk

½ cup water

2 eggs

3 tablespoons melted coconut oil

1 cup shredded cheddar cheese

Preparation Method

- ✓ Heat up your waffle iron.
- ✓ Mix together the flour, baking powder, and seasonings.
- ✓ Add the wet ingredients and form a batter.
- ✓ Add the cheese and mix together once more.
- ✓ Grease the waffle pan and scoop some of the mixture inside.
- ✓ Repeat until you have cooked the whole batch.
- ✓ Serve with honey or butter

Nutritional information

- ✓ Fat per serving – 17 grams
- ✓ Net carbs per serving – 3.81 grams
- ✓ Protein per serving – 6.52 grams
- ✓ Calories per serving – 214 calories

Crack Slaw Salad, Keto Style!

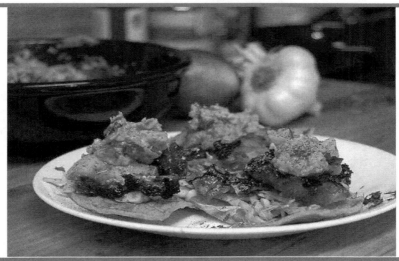

Category – Salads Servings – 4	Cooking time – 5 min Preparation time - 20 min

Ingredients

2 garlic cloves

2 tablespoons sesame seed oil

1 pound ground beef

10 ounces coleslaw salad mixture

1 tablespoon sriracha sauce

1 tablespoon soy sauce

1 teaspoon vinegar

¼ teaspoon black pepper

1/2 teaspoon Himalayan sea salt

1 teaspoon sesame seeds

1 stalk of a green onion

Preparation Method

- ✓ Heat up the sesame oil in a large wok.
- ✓ Crush the garlic cloves and cook in the oil.
- ✓ Brown the meat.
- ✓ Add the coleslaw mixture and combine with the cooked meat.
- ✓ Add the sriracha, soy sauce, vinegar and combine.
- ✓ Cook for 5 minutes.
- ✓ Season and serve.

Nutritional information

- ✓ Fat per serving – 27 grams
- ✓ Net carbs per serving – 4 grams
- ✓ Protein per serving – 24 grams
- ✓ Calories per serving – 350 calories

Grilled Cheese Sandwich

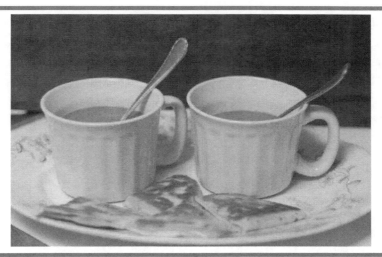

| Category – Breackfast/Lunch | Cooking time – 15 min |
| Servings – 1 | Preparation time - 5 min |

Ingredients

2 eggs

2 tablespoons almond flour

1 1/2 tablespoons psyllium husk powder

½ teaspoon baking powder

2 tablespoons softened butter,

2 ounces cheddar cheese

1 tablespoon butter

Preparation Method

- ✓ Soften the butter to room temperature and add the almond flour, psyllium husk and baking powder.
- ✓ Combine all together to make a dough.
- ✓ Add the eggs and combine.
- ✓ Place the mixture into a container, preferably square.
- ✓ Microwave for 90 seconds.
- ✓ Cut the bread in half.
- ✓ Divide the cheese between halves of bread.
- ✓ Melt 1 tablespoon of butter over a medium heat.
- ✓ Cook the sandwich on both sides.

Nutritional information

- ✓ Fat per serving – 70 grams
- ✓ Net carbs per serving – 4.7 grams
- ✓ Protein per serving – 29 grams
- ✓ Calories per serving – 793 calories

Avocado Tuna Melts

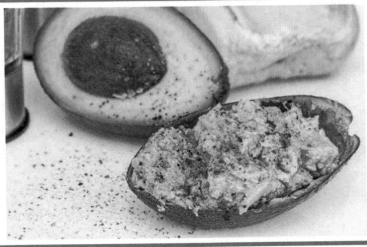

Category – Lunch/Snacks Servings – 12	Cooking time – 15 min Preparation time - 15 min

Ingredients

10 ounces canned tuna

¼ cup mayonnaise

1 avocado, cubed

¼ cup parmesan cheese

1/3 cup almond flour

½ teaspoon garlic powder

¼ teaspoon onion powder

Salt

Pepper

½ cup coconut oil

Preparation Method

- ✓ Drain the tuna and empty into a large bowl.
- ✓ Combine with the mayonnaise, spices, and parmesan.
- ✓ Slice the avocado in half and cube the inside.
- ✓ Add the avocado cubes to the mixture and combine.
- ✓ Form the mixture together into balls and roll in almond flour.
- ✓ Heat up the coconut oil over a medium heat.
- ✓ Fry the balls on all sides until golden.
- ✓ Serve!

Nutritional information

- ✓ Fat per serving – 11.8 grams
- ✓ Net carbs per serving – 0.8 grams
- ✓ Protein per serving – 6.2 grams
- ✓ Calories per serving – 135 calories

Stuffed Mushrooms

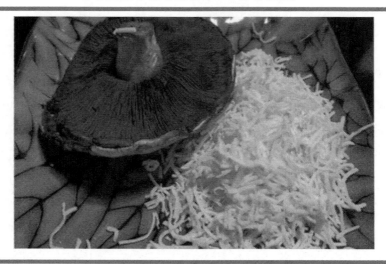

| Category – Lunch/Snacks | Cooking time – 10 min |
| Servings – 1 | Preparation time - 10 min |

Ingredients

2 Portobello or cremini mushrooms

1 clove garlic

¼ teaspoon Italian seasoning

Spinach

2 slices bacon

Cheese

Preparation Method

- ✓ Bake the bacon in the oven until crispy.

- ✓ Crumble the bacon once cooked.

- ✓ De-stalk the mushrooms.

- ✓ Mix together the cheese, seasonings, spinach, and bacon.

- ✓ Stuff the mushroom with the mixture.

- ✓ Bake in the oven until melted and cooked.

Nutritional information

- ✓ Fat per serving – 9 grams

- ✓ Net carbs per serving – 4.2 grams

- ✓ Protein per serving – 9.9 grams

- ✓ Calories per serving – 153 calories

Hot Chocolate

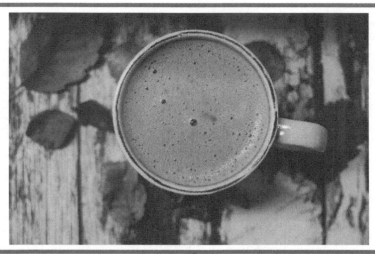

Category – Snacks	Cooking time – 5 min
Servings – 1	Preparation time - 10 min

Ingredients

1 cup coconut almond milk

Dagoba 73% Cacao Chocodrops

15 chips

½ teaspoon coconut oil

1 tablespoon heavy cream

Preparation Method

✓ Bring the coconut almond milk to a simmer and add in the chocolate chips to melt – stir continually.

✓ Add the coconut oil and keep stirring.

✓ Pour the mixture into a mug.

✓ Top with heavy cream and combine.

✓ Mix together.

✓ Enjoy!

Nutritional information

✓ Fat per serving – 9 grams

✓ Net carbs per serving – 3 grams

✓ Protein per serving – 1 grams

✓ Calories per serving – 103 calories

Chapter 7 30 to 60 Minute Recipes

We've covered mostly snacks, soups, salads, breakfast, and lunch recipes so far, but now we're going to move into recipes which take a little more time to prepare and cook. These recipes are therefore ideal for dinner, with a few other category options thrown in for good measure.

One Pan Chicken Thighs

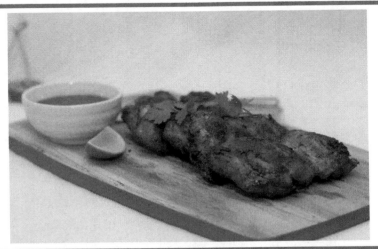

| Category – Dinner | Cooking time – 30 min |
| Servings – 4 | Preparation time - 10 min |

Ingredients

4 boneless chicken thighs

2 zucchini, sliced

½ cup sliced carrot

1 cup daikon radish

¼ cup olive oil

2 tablespoons balsamic vinegar

1 tablespoon minced ginger

Preparation Method

- ✓ Preheat the oven to 350°F.
- ✓ Place the chicken thighs on a greased baking dish.
- ✓ Cut up the zucchini, carrot, and radish into slices, place around the chicken.
- ✓ Combine the olive oil, balsamic vinegar, and ginger.
- ✓ Pour over the chicken and season.
- ✓ Cook for half an hour.

Nutritional information

- ✓ Fat per serving – 12 grams
- ✓ Net carbs per serving – 9 grams
- ✓ Protein per serving – 8 grams
- ✓ Calories per serving – 437 calories

Ham, Cheddar & Chive Soufflé

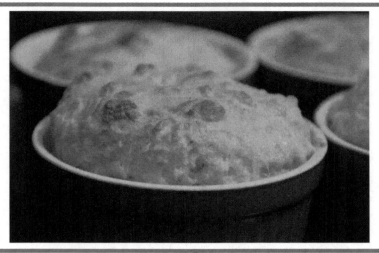

Category – Dinner/Lunch	Cooking time – 20 min
Servings – 1	Preparation time - 20 min

Ingredients

3 tablespoons olive oil

½ diced onion

½ teaspoon minced garlic

6 ounces cooked ham steak, cubed

1 tablespoon butter

6 eggs

1 cup shredded cheddar cheese

½ cup heavy cream

2-3 tablespoons chopped fresh chives

½ teaspoon salt

¼ teaspoon black pepper

Preparation Method

- ✓ Preheat the oven to 400°F.
- ✓ Dice and chop the onion, garlic, ham steak, and chives.
- ✓ Warm up the olive oil over a medium heat, cooking the onions until soft.
- ✓ Add the garlic.
- ✓ Add the eggs, cream, chopped chives, salt and pepper – mix together.
- ✓ Add the rest of the ingredients and mix together.
- ✓ Place the mixture into small muffin trays.
- ✓ Bake for 20 minutes.

Nutritional information

- ✓ Fat per serving – 39.6 grams
- ✓ Net carbs per serving – 3.5 grams
- ✓ Protein per serving – 19.6 grams
- ✓ Calories per serving – 404 calories

Chocolate Peanut Butter Muffins

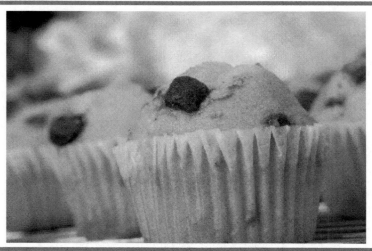

Category – Snacks/Dessert	Cooking time – 15 min
Servings – 1	Preparation time - 20 min

Ingredients

1 cup almond flour

1/2 cup erythritol

1 teaspoon baking powder

1 pinch salt

1/3 cup peanut butter

1/3 cup almond milk

2 eggs

½ cup sugar free chocolate chips

Preparation Method

✓ Preheat the oven to 350°F.

✓ Combine all the dry ingredients, but keep the chocolate chips to one side.

✓ Add the peanut butter and almond milk, and combine.

✓ Add one egg and stir, then repeat until eggs are gone.

✓ Fold in the chocolate chips evenly and carefully.

✓ Divide the mixture into a muffin tray.

✓ Bake for 15 minutes in the oven.

✓ Allow to cool.

Nutritional information

✓ Fat per serving – 41 grams

✓ Net carbs per serving – 4.5 grams

✓ Protein per serving – 15 grams

✓ Calories per serving – 530 calories

Broccoli and Cheddar Soup

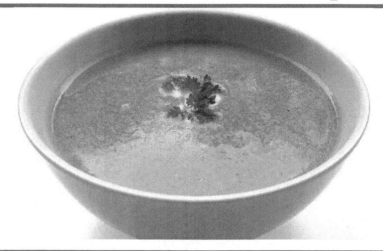

Category – Soup/Dinner	Cooking time – 25 min
Servings – 4	Preparation time - 25 min

Ingredients

1 tablespoon butter

½ onion

1 cup heavy cream

2 cups broth

2 cups water

12 ounces broccoli

8 ounces cheddar cheese

Salt

Pepper

½ teaspoon paprika

¼ teaspoon xanthan gum

Preparation Method

- ✓ Heat a large soup pot; melt the butter.

- ✓ Sauté the onion and garlic in the butter.

- ✓ Add the cream, broth, and water, and bring to the boil.

- ✓ Season the mixture with salt, pepper, and paprika.

- ✓ Add the broccoli florets to the mixture, and bring the temperature down to a simmer.

- ✓ Cook for 25 minutes.

- ✓ Add the cheddar cheese and stir well.

- ✓ Pour the mixture into a blender and blend until smooth.

- ✓ While you are blending, add a little xanthan gum at a time until you achieve the desired consistency.

- ✓ Pour into a dish and add a little cheese on top.

Nutritional information

- ✓ Fat per serving – 32 grams

- ✓ Net carbs per serving – 8 grams

- ✓ Protein per serving – 11 grams

- ✓ Calories per serving – 370 calories

Bacon, Avocado and Chicken Sandwich

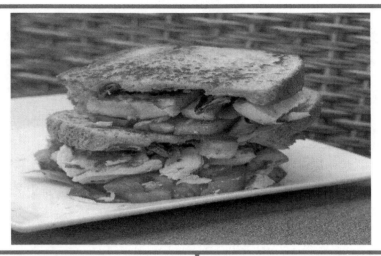

Category – Dinner/Lunch Servings – 2	Cooking time – 25 min Preparation time - 20 min

Ingredients

3 eggs

3 ounces cream cheese

1/8 teaspoon cream of tartar

¼ teaspoon salt

½ teaspoon garlic powder

1 tablespoon mayonnaise

1 teaspoon sriracha

2 slices bacon

3 ounces chicken

2 slices pepper jack cheese

2 cherry tomatoes

¼ avocado

Preparation Method

- ✓ Preheat the oven to 300°F.
- ✓ Separate the three eggs into two different bowls – whites and yolks separate.
- ✓ Add the cream of tartar to the whites and whisk.
- ✓ Add the cream cheese to the yolks and beat.
- ✓ Fold the half the whites into the yolks, and repeat for the rest.
- ✓ Place parchment onto a baking tray.
- ✓ Pour the mixture onto the paper into large circles and make a square.
- ✓ Sprinkle with garlic powder.
- ✓ Bake for 25 minutes.
- ✓ Cook the chicken and bacon in a skillet.
- ✓ Mix the mayonnaise and sriracha.
- ✓ Spread the mixture onto one side of the bread, and place the chicken on top.
- ✓ Add two slices of cheese and bacon, and halved tomatoes.
- ✓ Spread avocado mash on top and season.
- ✓ Put the 'lid' of the bread on top and serve.

Nutritional information

- ✓ Fat per serving – 28.3 grams
- ✓ Net carbs per serving – 2 grams
- ✓ Protein per serving – 22 grams
- ✓ Calories per serving – 361 calories

Sesame Chicken

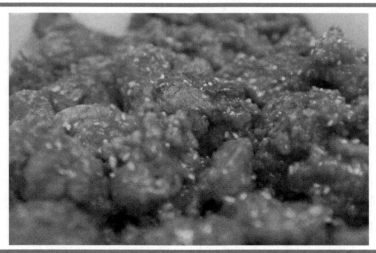

Category – Dinner Servings – 2	Cooking time – 25 min Preparation time - 5 min

Ingredients

1 egg

1 tablespoon arrowroot powder or corn starch

1 pound chicken thighs

2 tablespoons toasted sesame seed oil (1 tablespoon for chicken, 1 tablespoon for sauce)

Salt

Pepper

2 tablespoon soy sauce

2 tablespoon Sukrin Gold

1 tablespoon vinegar

1 centimeter cubed ginger

1 clove garlic

2 tablespoons sesame seeds

¼ teaspoon xanthan gum

Preparation Method

✓ Combine the arrowroot powder, corn starch and the egg.

✓ Coat the chicken in the mixture.

✓ Heat up the sesame seed oil and add the chicken, turning occasionally until cooked.

✓ Mix together the soy sauce, Sukrin Gold, ginger, garlic, xanthan gum, sesame seeds, and vinegar together.

✓ After the chicken is cooked, add the sauce to the same pan and stir for five minutes.

✓ Serve with extra sesame seeds.

Nutritional information

✓ Fat per serving – 36 grams

✓ Net carbs per serving – 4 grams

✓ Protein per serving – 45 grams

✓ Calories per serving – 520 calories

Chicken Kiev

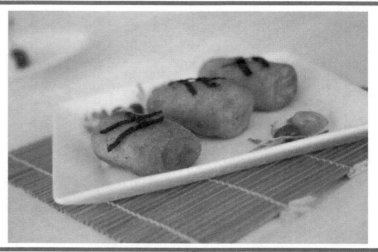

Category – Dinner	Cooking time – 20 min
Servings – 2	Preparation time - 30 min

Ingredients

2 chicken breasts

4 tablespoons butter

2 cloves garlic

1 stalk green onion

Tarragon

Parsley

Salt

Pepper

1 ounce pork rinds

1 egg

¼ cup coconut flour

Preparation Method

✓ Preheat the oven to 350°F.

✓ Season the chicken with parsley, tarragon, salt, and pepper, to taste.

✓ Spread the butter on top of the chicken breast, the onion and chopped garlic.

✓ Roll up the chicken and hold together with toothpicks.

✓ Crush the pork rinds in a blender.

✓ Place the coconut flour in one bowl, the beaten egg in another, and the pork rinds in a third bowl.

✓ First, dip the chicken into the flour, then into the egg, and then into the pork rinds – the chicken should be completely coated in all three.

✓ Refrigerate for 30 minutes.

✓ Fry the chicken on all sides.

✓ Put the chicken into a baking dish and bake for 20 minutes.

✓ Serve

Nutritional information

✓ Fat per serving – 33 grams

✓ Net carbs per serving – 4 grams

✓ Protein per serving – 50 grams

✓ Calories per serving – 510 calories

Cheddar, Chicken and Broccoli Casserole

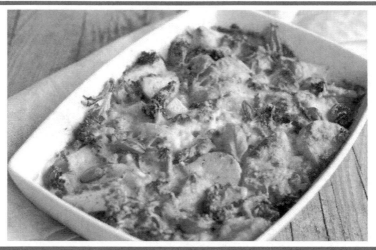

Category – Dinner Servings – 6	Cooking time – 25 min Preparation time - 30 min

Ingredients

20 ounces chicken breast

2 tablespoons olive oil

2 cups broccoli

½ cup sour cream

½ cup heavy cream

1 cup cheddar cheese

1 ounce pork rinds

Salt

Pepper

½ teaspoon paprika

1 teaspoon oregano

Preparation Method

- ✓ Preheat the oven to 450°F.

- ✓ Shred the cooked chicken breast into pieces.

- ✓ Mix together the chicken, broccoli, olive oil and sour cream, mix together to make sure all combined.

- ✓ Grease a large baking dish and place the mixture inside.

- ✓ Pour the heavy cream over the top and season.

- ✓ Add the cheddar cheese. Crush the pork rinds down with a rolling pin and sprinkle over the dish as the last layer.

- ✓ Bake in the oven for 20-25 minutes.

Nutritional information

- ✓ Fat per serving – 28 grams

- ✓ Net carbs per serving – 2.6 grams

- ✓ Protein per serving – 29 grams

- ✓ Calories per serving – 365 calories

Nacho Chicken Casserole

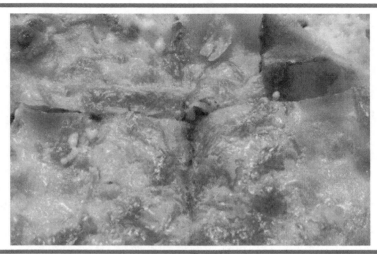

Category – Dinner	Cooking time – 20 min
Servings – 6	Preparation time - 25 min

Ingredients

1 ¾ pounds boneless, skinless chicken thighs

1 ½ teaspoon chili seasoning

2 tablespoons olive oil

4 ounces cream cheese

4 ounces cheddar cheese

1 cup green chilies and tomatoes

3 tablespoons parmesan cheese

¼ cup sour cream

16 ounces pack of frozen cauliflower

1 jalapeno pepper

Salt

Pepper

Preparation Method

- ✓ Preheat the oven to 375°F.
- ✓ Cut the chicken into chunks and season.
- ✓ Brown the chicken over a medium heat.
- ✓ Add the cream cheese, sour cream and cheddar cheese and mix.
- ✓ Add the tomatoes and green chilies.
- ✓ Transfer to a baking dish.
- ✓ Cut the jalapeno into pieces.
- ✓ Spread the cauliflower over the top of the baking dish mixture and sprinkle the pepper over the top.
- ✓ Bake in the oven for 15-20 minutes.

Nutritional information

- ✓ Fat per serving – 32.2 grams
- ✓ Net carbs per serving – 4.3 grams
- ✓ Protein per serving – 30.8 grams
- ✓ Calories per serving – 426 calories

Keto Pizza

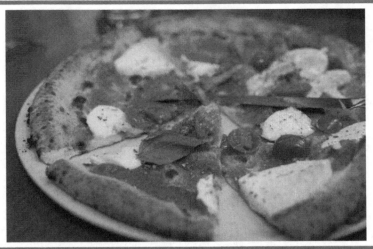

Category – Dinner Servings – 1	Cooking time – 20 min Preparation time - 10 min

Ingredients

2 eggs

2 tablespoons parmesan cheese

1 tablespoon psyllium husk powder

½ tsp Italian seasoning

Salt

2 teaspoons frying oil

1 ½ ounces mozzarella cheese

3 tablespoons tomato sauce

1 tablespoons chopped basil

Preparation Method

- ✓ Place the parmesan, psyllium husk powder, Italian seasoning and salt into a blender with two eggs and blend.
- ✓ Heat a large frying pan and add the oil.
- ✓ Add the mixture to the pan in a large circular shape.
- ✓ Flip once the underside is browning and then remove from pan.
- ✓ Spoon the tomato sauce onto the pizza crust and spread.
- ✓ Add the cheese and spread over the top of the pizza.
- ✓ Place the pizza into the oven – it is finished once the cheese is melted.

Nutritional information

- ✓ Fat per serving – 35 grams
- ✓ Net carbs per serving – 3.5 grams
- ✓ Protein per serving – 27 grams
- ✓ Calories per serving – 459 calories

Chicken Curry

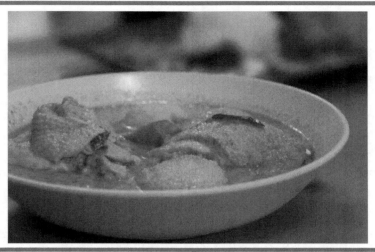

Category – Dinner	Cooking time – 20 min
Servings – 3	Preparation time - 20 min

Ingredients

2 tablespoons coconut oil

1 ½ inch ginger

1 green chili

2 shallots

2 cloves garlic

2 teaspoons turmeric powder

1 stalk lemongrass

½ cup coconut milk

½ cup water

6 chicken drumsticks

½ teaspoon salt

1 tablespoon cilantro, chopped

Preparation Method

- ✓ Bruise the lemongrass to bring the flavor out.
- ✓ Using a pestle and mortar, combine the ginger, green chilli, shallots, and garlic.
- ✓ Melt the coconut oil in a large pot.
- ✓ Add the ingredients and sauté.
- ✓ After a few minutes add the turmeric powder and lemongrass.
- ✓ Add the chicken and continue cooking.
- ✓ Pour in half a cup of coconut milk and half a cup of water.
- ✓ Add the salt.
- ✓ Cover the pot.
- ✓ Cook for 20 minutes – check the chicken is cooked properly.
- ✓ Serve with chopped cilantro.

Nutritional information

- ✓ Fat per serving – 35 grams
- ✓ Net carbs per serving – 4.8 grams
- ✓ Protein per serving – 37.5 grams
- ✓ Calories per serving – 493 calories

Walnut Crusted Salmon

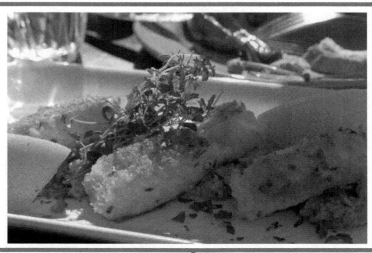

Category – Dinner Servings – 2	Cooking time – 15 min Preparation time - 15 min

Ingredients

½ cup walnuts

2 tablespoons sugar free maple syrup

1/2 tablespoons Dijon mustard

¼ teaspoon dill

2/3 ounce salmon fillets

1 tablespoon olive oil

4 or 5 spinach leaves

Salt

Pepper

Preparation Method

- ✓ Preheat the oven to 350°F.
- ✓ In a food processor, pulse together the walnuts, maple syrup and spices, then add the mustard.
- ✓ Heat the oil on a medium heat using a large skillet.
- ✓ With the skin side down, fry the salmon fillets for around three minutes.
- ✓ Add the mixture onto the top of the fish.
- ✓ Once the underside is cooked, bake in the oven for 8 minutes.
- ✓ Serve over the spinach.

Nutritional information

- ✓ Fat per serving – 43 grams
- ✓ Net carbs per serving – 3 grams
- ✓ Protein per serving – 20 grams
- ✓ Calories per serving – 373 calories

Coconut Chicken Tenders

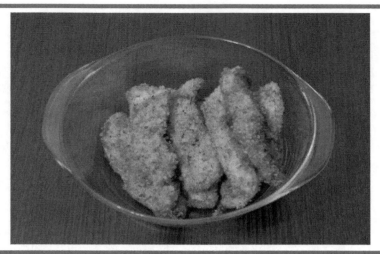

Category – Dinner Servings – 4	Cooking time – 20 min Preparation time - 5 min

Ingredients

1 pound boneless and skinless chicken tenders

1 egg

½ cup cashew flour

1 cup shredded coconut

¼ teaspoon salt

¼ teaspoon pepper

¼ teaspoon garlic powder

1/8 teaspoon cinnamon

Preparation Method

- ✓ Preheat the oven to 375°F.

- ✓ Beat the egg and set aside.

- ✓ In a separate bowl, combine the cashew flour, the coconut and the spices.

- ✓ Dip each chicken tender, first in the egg, and then the coconut spice batter.

- ✓ Place each tender on a pan lined with baking parchment.

- ✓ Bake in the oven for around 20 minutes, or until cooked.

Nutritional information

- ✓ Fat per serving – 6.7 grams

- ✓ Net carbs per serving – 16.7 grams

- ✓ Protein per serving – 28.8 grams

- ✓ Calories per serving – 242 calories

Pizza Frittata

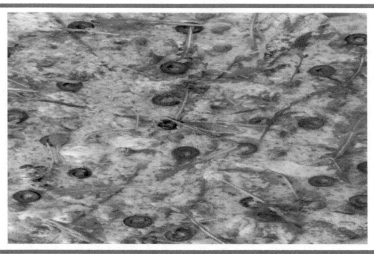

Category – Breakfast/Lunch Servings – 8	Cooking time – 30 min Preparation time - 15 min

Ingredients

12 eggs

9 ounce bag frozen spinach

1 ounce pepperoni

5 ounces mozzarella cheese

1 teaspoon garlic, minced

½ cup ricotta cheese

½ cup parmesan cheese,

4 tablespoon olive oil

1/4 teaspoon nutmeg

Salt

Pepper

Preparation Method

✓ Microwave the spinach on defrost.

✓ Preheat your oven to 375°F.

✓ Combine the ricotta, the parmesan and spinach.

✓ Pour the mixture into a baking dish.

✓ Sprinkle the mozzarella over the mixture.

✓ Add the pepperoni.

✓ Bake for half an hour, until set.

Nutritional information

✓ Fat per serving – 23.8 grams

✓ Net carbs per serving – 2.1 grams

✓ Protein per serving – 19.4 grams

✓ Calories per serving – 298 calories

Chapter 8 Pressure Cooker Recipes

Creating meals with a pressure cooker is a big deal these days. In fact, you could argue that it's fashionable. The fact you are following the keto diet doesn't mean you can't get in on this fast cooking trend; in fact, it's encouraged. You're using fresh, clean ingredients, so there's no reduction of taste or nutrition by using a pressure cooker.

Pressure Cooker Tomato Sauce

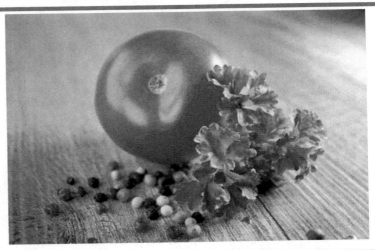

Category – *Sauces/Dressings* Servings – Large batch, one serving is ¼ cup	Cooking time – 1 h 15 min Preparation time - 15 min

Ingredients

4 tablespoons olive oil
2 sliced yellow onions
2 chopped carrots
1 chopped celery stalk
6 pounds quartered plum tomatoes
6 fresh basil leaves

Preparation Method

- ✓ Preheat your pressure cooker and add the oil and onion; sauté until soft.
- ✓ Slice the tomatoes.
- ✓ Add the carrots and celery to the cooker and sauté for 5 minutes.
- ✓ Add the tomatoes and mix well .
- ✓ Bring the cooker to the boil, using the sauté mode.
- ✓ Close the lid and cook at high pressure for 5 minutes.
- ✓ Open the cooker and mix the contents, allowing it to simmer on a low heat for 1 hour, until the contents have reduced down to around half.
- ✓ Combine the contents with an immersion blender.
- ✓ Pour into jars and store.

Nutritional information

- ✓ Fat per serving – 2.1 grams
- ✓ Net carbs per serving – 3.2 grams
- ✓ Protein per serving – 1 grams
- ✓ Calories per serving – 42.9 calories

Black Bean & Lentil Chilli

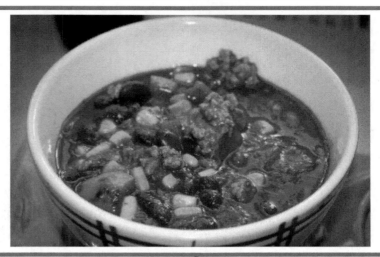

Category – Dinner	Cooking time – 15 min
Servings – 6	Preparation time - 5 min

Ingredients

1 tablespoon olive oil

2 chopped carrots

1 tablespoon paprika

1 tablespoon dried oregano

2 teaspoons garlic powder

2 teaspoons cumin

1 ounce dried mushrooms

1 cup lentils

2 cups dry black beans

1 14 ounce can of chopped tomatoes

4 cups of water

2 tablespoons Worcestershire sauce

1 teaspoon salt

Preparation Method

✓ Preheat your pressure cooker using a 'sauté' or 'brown' program.

✓ Chop the onions and the carrot.

✓ Add the oil and onion to the pressure cooker.

✓ Add the spices, mushrooms, carrots and tomatoes, mix well.

✓ Close the lid and set the pressure cooker valve for 10 minutes on high.

✓ Add the salt.

✓ Add the Worcestershire sauce and combine.

✓ Serve in a bowl.

Nutritional information

✓ Fat per serving – 2.5 grams

✓ Net carbs per serving – 4.2 grams

✓ Protein per serving – 8 grams

✓ Calories per serving – 144.9 calories

Eggplant and Olive Spread

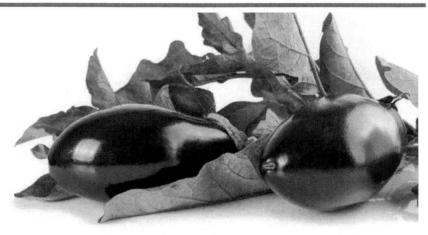

Category – Snack Servings – 6	Cooking time – 5 min Preparation time - 2 min

Ingredients

4 tablespoons olive oil

2 pounds eggplant

3 garlic cloves (skin on)

1 teaspoon salt

½ cup water

1 lemon juiced

1 tablespoon tahini

¼ cup black pitted olives

Thyme, a few sprigs

Extra virgin olive oil

Preparation Method

✓ Peel the eggplant and slice into big chunks to cover the bottom of your pressure cooker.

✓ Preheat your cooker to medium heat and leave the lid off.

✓ Add the olive oil to the cooker and then add the eggplant once hot – these chunks will caramelise on one side only.

✓ After 5 minutes, add the garlic cloves.

✓ Turn the eggplant to cook on the other side.

✓ Add the rest of the eggplant, salt, and water.

✓ Close the pressure cooker and cook for 3 minutes on high pressure.

✓ Remove the garlic cloves and take off the skin.

✓ Add the tahini, lemon juice, garlic cloves, olives and puree with an immersion blender.

✓ Sprinkle with fresh thyme and olive oil.

Nutritional information

✓ Fat per serving – 11.7 grams

✓ Net carbs per serving – 7 grams

✓ Protein per serving – 2 grams

✓ Calories per serving – 155.5 calories

BBQ Sauce

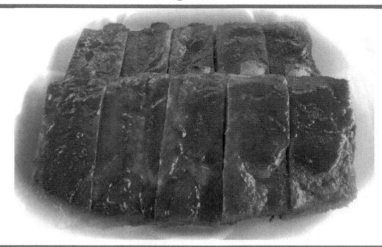

| Category – Snack/dressing | Cooking time – 15 min |
| Servings – 2 | Preparation time - 5 min |

Ingredients

1 tablespoon sesame seed oil

1 chopped medium onion

½ cup tomato puree or passata

½ cup water

4 tablespoons honey

4 tablespoons white vinegar

1 teaspoon sea salt

½ teaspoon garlic powder

1 teaspoon hot sauce

1 teaspoon liquid smoke

1/8 teaspoon ground clove powder

1/8 teaspoon cumin powder

¾ cup seedless dried plums (prunes)

Preparation Method

✓ Preheat your pressure cooker.

✓ Add the sesame oil and onion and sauté, stirring every so often.

✓ In a 2 cup measuring cup, add the tomato puree, water, honey, and vinegar. Combine and then add the salt, garlic, hot sauce, liquid smoke, clove, and cumin.

✓ Mix this all together well and ensure the honey is dissolved.

✓ Pour the mixture into the pressure cooker.

✓ Add the plums.

✓ Close the lid and cook for 10 minutes on high pressure.

✓ Once finished, use an immersion blender to puree everything together.

Nutritional information

✓ Fat per serving – 0.4 grams

✓ Net carbs per serving – 2.8 grams

✓ Protein per serving – 0.1 grams

✓ Calories per serving – 20.3 calories

Split Pea & Smoky Pancetta Soup

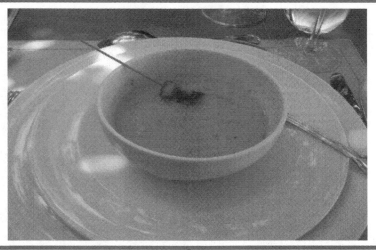

Category – Soup Servings – 6	Cooking time – 15 min Preparation time - 10 min

Ingredients

3.5 ounces bacon or smoked pancetta

1 diced medium onion

1 diced celery stalk

1 diced carrot

2 cups dried green split peas

6 cups of water

1 bay leaf

1 teaspoon sea salt

Preparation Method

- ✓ To your cold pressure cooker, add the bacon or pancetta and heat to medium.
- ✓ Once the meat begins to fry, stir and allow it to crisp and then remove from the heat.
- ✓ Add the onion, celery and carrot to the cooker and sauté them in the fat until the onion browns.
- ✓ Add the split peas, water, bay leaf, and salt, and combine together well – the pressure cooker should be only half full.
- ✓ Close the lid and cook for 5 minutes at high pressure.
- ✓ Open the lid and mix the soup.
- ✓ Serve with the rest of the pancetta as a garnish.

Nutritional information

- ✓ Fat per serving – 7.6 grams
- ✓ Net carbs per serving – 4.8 grams
- ✓ Protein per serving – 8.5 grams
- ✓ Calories per serving – 171.5 calories

Steamed Artichokes

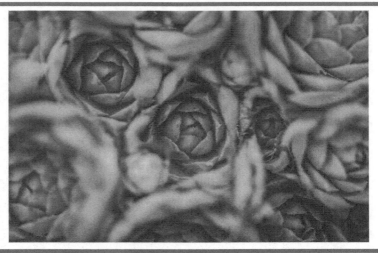

Category – Dinner Servings – 4	Cooking time – 15 min Preparation time - 10 min

Ingredients

2 medium artichokes

1 lemon (in halves)

2 tablespoons mayonnaise

1 teaspoon Dijon mustard

1 pinch of paprika

Preparation Method

✓ Trim the artichokes and remove the outer leaves. Wipe the edges with half a lemon.

✓ Now you need to steam the artichokes – add a cup of water to your pressure cooker and place inside using the basket, artichokes facing upward. Add the lemon juice again.

✓ Close the lid and cook for 10 minutes at high pressure.

✓ Open the lid and move from the burner to cool.

✓ If the leaf is easy to remove from the artichoke, it is cooked.

✓ Mix mayonnaise and mustard together in a bowl and sprinkle in the paprika.

✓ Serve together while still warm.

Nutritional information

✓ Fat per serving – 5 grams

✓ Net carbs per serving – 3.5 grams

✓ Protein per serving – 2 grams

✓ Calories per serving – 77.5 calories

Lentil Risotto

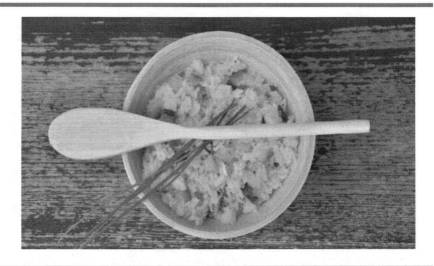

Category – Lunch/Dinner Servings – 6	Cooking time – 10 min Preparation time - 10 min

Ingredients

1 cup dry lentils (soaked the night before)

1 tablespoon olive oil

1 chopped onion (medium)

1 stalk chopped celery

2 sprigs parsley, chopped

1 cup Arborio rice

2 garlic cloves

3 ¼ cups vegetable stock

Preparation Method

- ✓ Preheat your pressure cooker and then add the olive oil.
- ✓ Add the onion and sauté until soft.
- ✓ Add the celery, parsley, and sauté for one minute.
- ✓ Add the rice and garlic cloves and sauté for another minute.
- ✓ Add the stock and lentils – mix together.
- ✓ Close the lid and cook on high pressure for 5 minutes.
- ✓ Mix well and serve immediately.

Nutritional information

- ✓ Fat per serving – 2.5 grams
- ✓ Net carbs per serving – 2.1 grams
- ✓ Protein per serving – 5.7 grams
- ✓ Calories per serving – 190 calories

Chicken Cacciatore with Burst Cherry Tomatoes

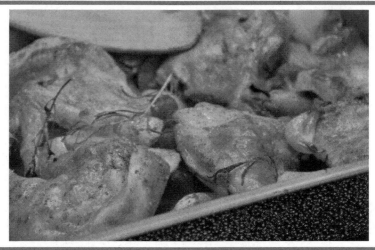

Category – Dinner	Cooking time – 30 min
Servings – 6	Preparation time - 10 min

Ingredients

1 /2 pound chicken breasts, skinless and boneless

1 pound cherry tomatoes

2 garlic cloves, crushed

1 cup water

½ cup pitted green olives

¼ cup red wine (tart flavor)

1 teaspoon olive oil

1 teaspoon kosher salt

1 teaspoon dried oregano

1 spring fresh basil

¼ teaspoon hot pepper flakes

Preparation Method

✓ Heat your pressure cooker with the oil.

✓ Once hot, add the chicken breasts and brown on both sides.

✓ Place the cherry tomatoes into a plastic bag and tie – crush the tomatoes until they are open, but not squashed.

✓ Remove the chicken from the pressure cooker and pour in the tomatoes and juice.

✓ Add the hot pepper flakes, salt, wine, water, oregano, garlic, and mix together.

✓ Add the chicken back into the cooker and stir it around to coat.

✓ Close the lid and cook on high pressure for 12 minutes.

✓ Stir and rest for 5 minutes.

✓ Serve with green olives and basil

Nutritional information

✓ Fat per serving – 6.4 grams

✓ Net carbs per serving – 6.6 grams

✓ Protein per serving – 4.3 grams

✓ Calories per serving – 81.3 calories

Tomatillo Chilli

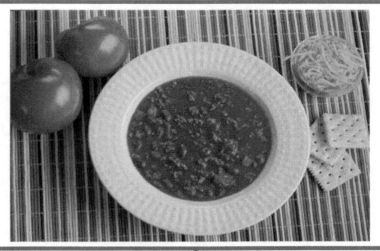

Category – Lunch/Dinner Servings – 6	Cooking time – 40 min Preparation time - 10 min

Ingredients

1 pound ground beef

1 pound ground pork

3 medium chopped tomatillos

½ chopped onion

6 ounces tomato paste

1 teaspoon garlic powder

1 jalapeno pepper, including seeds

1 tablespoon ground cumin

1 tablespoon chilli powder

¼ cup water

Salt

Preparation Method

✓ Heat the pressure cooker and use it to brown the meats.

✓ Add the other ingredients to the pressure cooker and stir together.

✓ Close the cooker and cook on high pressure for 35 minutes.

✓ Remove from heat and allow to rest.

✓ Remove the lid and stir.

✓ Serve!

Nutritional information

✓ Fat per serving – 35.8 grams

✓ Net carbs per serving – 5.47 grams

✓ Protein per serving – 22.3 grams

✓ Calories per serving – 443.4 calories

BBQ Pork Ribs with Spinach Bean Salad

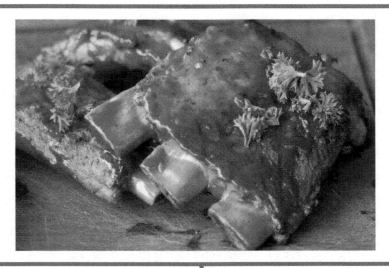

Category – Dinner	Cooking time – 30 min
Servings – 6	Preparation time - 15 min

Ingredients

1 ½ pounds baby back pork ribs

1 cup barbecue sauce

1 pinch salt

1 pinch ground black pepper

1 tablespoon olive oil

1 diced onion

1 ½ cups water

1 cup dried cannellini beans

1 bay leaf

1 finely chopped garlic clove

6 ounces fresh spinach

Preparation Method

- ✓ Cut the ribs apart and coat them with the barbecue sauce on all sides.
- ✓ Sprinkle the ribs with salt and pepper and place into the steamer basket – set aside.
- ✓ Heat the pressure cooker on medium heat and add the oil.
- ✓ Stir in the onion and sauté until soft.
- ✓ Add the water, beans, bay leaf, and stir.
- ✓ Lower the steamer basket containing the ribs into the pressure cooker and close. Cook for 20 minutes on high pressure.
- ✓ Place the lid of the pressure cooker on your countertop upside-down and lift the steamer basket out of the pressure cooker. Place the basket on the lid
- ✓ Remove the bay leaf and throw away.
- ✓ Mix in 1 teaspoon salt, garlic and the spinach.
- ✓ Spoon the bean mixture into a large casserole dish which is big enough to hold the ribs all in one layer.
- ✓ Arrange the ribs on top of the bean mixture and brush with what is left of the barbeque sauce.
- ✓ Broil the casserole until the sauce is caramelised.
- ✓ Serve immediately.

Nutritional information

- ✓ Fat per serving – 39.5 grams
- ✓ Net carbs per serving – 8.2 grams
- ✓ Protein per serving – 33.6 grams
- ✓ Calories per serving – 572 calories

Pork & Hominy Stew

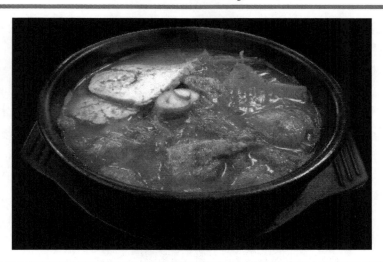

Category – Dinner	Cooking time – 45 min
Servings – 6	Preparation time - 10 min

Ingredients

2 cups dry hominy kernels, soaked overnight

4 cups water

2 pounds boneless pork, sliced into two chunks

2 bay leaves

2 dried ancho chilies

1 teaspoon dried Mexican oregano

1 teaspoon 0.

cumin powder

3 cloves garlic

3 teaspoons salt

1 fresh red bell pepper

Preparation Method

- ✓ Add the soaked hominy and the water to the pressure cooker.
- ✓ Cook on a high pressure at 15 minutes.
- ✓ Once cooked, open the lid and add the meat, bay leaves, dry ancho chilies, oregano, cumin, garlic, and salt.
- ✓ Close the lid and cook again on high pressure for 10 minutes.
- ✓ Open the lid and allow to rest for 10 minutes.
- ✓ Discard the bay leaf and remove the ancho chilies.
- ✓ Puree the chilies, two spoons of hominy from the cooker, fresh pepper, and garlic into a paste and put back into the pressure cooker.
- ✓ Simmer for 5-10 minutes.
- ✓ Serve

Nutritional information

- ✓ Fat per serving – 11.5 grams
- ✓ Net carbs per serving – 8.2 grams
- ✓ Protein per serving – 15.8 grams
- ✓ Calories per serving – 216.2 calories

Pressure Cooker Risotto

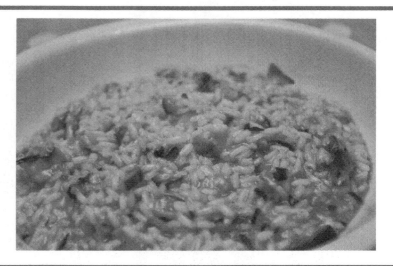

| Category – Lunch/Dinner | Cooking time – 15 min |
| Servings – 6 | Preparation time - 2 min |

Ingredients

2 cups Arborio rice

2 cups chicken or vegetable broth

1 chopped onion

1 dash of white wine

Extra virgin olive oil

1 tablespoon parmesan cheese

Salt

Pepper

Preparation Method

- ✓ Preheat your pressure cooker on a medium heat and then add the oil and onion.
- ✓ Sauté the onion until it is translucent.
- ✓ Add the rice and toast it lightly to release the starch content.
- ✓ Add the white wine and stir.
- ✓ Add the broth and mix – close the lid immediately.
- ✓ Close the cooker and cook on high pressure for 5-6 minutes.
- ✓ Stir. The rice will continue to absorb the liquid quite quickly.
- ✓ Stir in the cheese before serving.

Nutritional information

- ✓ Fat per serving – 5 grams
- ✓ Net carbs per serving – 6.2 grams
- ✓ Protein per serving – 12 grams
- ✓ Calories per serving – 339 calories

Buffalicious Chicken Wings

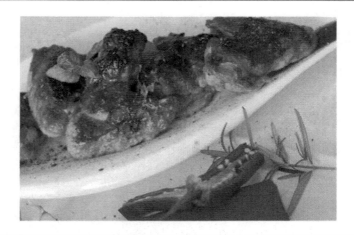

Category – Dinner	Cooking time – 25 min
Servings – 6	Preparation time - 5 min

Ingredients

2 pounds chicken wings

1 pound celery

4 tablespoons hot sauce

¼ cup honey

¼ cup tomato puree

3 teaspoon salt

1 cup plaint whole milk yogurt

1 tablespoon parsley

Preparation Method

- ✓ Prepare the pressure cooker with 1 cup of water and a steamer basket.
- ✓ Place the chicken wings evenly spaced in the steamer basket.
- ✓ Close the lid and cook for 10 minutes on high pressure.
- ✓ In a large bowl, add the hot sauce, honey, tomato puree, and salt.
- ✓ Mix the contents together until the honey is totally combined.
- ✓ When the chicken is cooked, coat it in the mixture and place the pieces on parchment paper.
- ✓ Slide under a broiler for 5 minutes until cooked and brown.
- ✓ Prepare your serving platter with celery sticks and yogurt.

Nutritional information

- ✓ Fat per serving – 8 grams
- ✓ Net carbs per serving – 8 grams
- ✓ Protein per serving – 17 grams
- ✓ Calories per serving – 180 calories

Egg Roll Soup

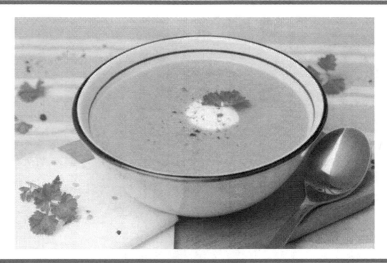

Category – Lunch/Dinner	Cooking time – 40 min
Servings – 6	Preparation time - 10 min

Ingredients

1 tablespoon ghee, olive oil, or avocado oil

1 pound ground pastured pork

1 diced onion

32 ounces chicken or beef broth

½ cabbage head, chopped

2 cups shredded carrots

1 teaspoon garlic powder

1 teaspoon onion powder

1 teaspoon sea salt

1 teaspoon ground ginger

2/3 cup coconut aminos

Preparation Method

✓ In your pressure cooker, brown the pork using 1 tablespoon of the cooking fat.

✓ Add the onion.

✓ Add the remaining ingredients and cook for 25 minutes on high pressure.

✓ Remove the lid and serve.

Nutritional information

✓ Fat per serving – 12.9 grams

✓ Net carbs per serving – 5.2 grams

✓ Protein per serving – 18.7 grams

✓ Calories per serving – 218 calories

Beef Stew

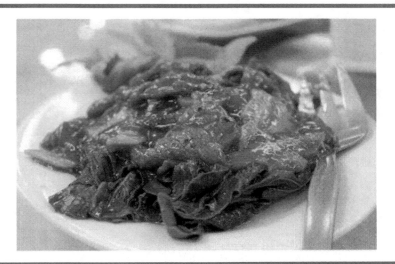

Category – Dinner	Cooking time – 40 min
Servings – 6	Preparation time - 10 min

Ingredients

2 pounds beef stew meat

2 tablespoons oil

1 sliced onion

4 peeled and sliced carrots

4 garlic cloves

3 cups of beef broth

1 cup water

1 tablespoon tomato paste

2 bay leaves

6 sprigs of thyme

Preparation Method

✓ Season the meat with salt and pepper.

✓ Heat the oil in the pressure cooker with the lid off, on a medium to high heat.

✓ Brown the meat for 3-5 minutes.

✓ Add the onion, carrots and garlic.

✓ Sauté and then add the broth, tomato paste, bay leaves, and thyme sprigs.

✓ Add the lid and turn the heat to high. Cook on high pressure for 25 minutes.

✓ Add salt and pepper.

Nutritional information

✓ Fat per serving – 5.7 grams

✓ Net carbs per serving – 2.7 grams

✓ Protein per serving – 8 grams

✓ Calories per serving – 86 calories

Conclusion

Are you ready and raring to go? The hope is that you're nodding 'yes'.

Throughout this book, we have given you all the help and advice we can, to push you toward overall health and well-being. Now it's up to you!

If we can leave you with one thought, it is this: Remember that the ketogenic diet is an overall lifestyle change. It is not something which you can plan to follow for a few weeks, lose the weight, and then go back to a 'normal' life. Ketosis is not something you should confuse your body with on a regular basis, because you could send your system into total shock. Ketosis needs to be introduced, acclimated to, and maintained. That is the only healthy way to enjoy the benefits of the keto diet. If you use it as a pick-up and set-down mechanism, it will have detrimental effects.

The great thing about this diet is that it gives you the choice to enjoy some delicious and healthy meals, using clean produce which is flavorful and tasty. Keto foods are packed with those vitamins and minerals we need for overall health and well-being. When you add exercise into the mix, perhaps with a friend to make it a fun, social experience, you have a lifestyle package. This package can revolutionize not only the way you eat, but how you feel on the inside and outside, too.

What more is there to say? Good luck you with your keto endeavours. This is one step you won't regret taking!

My other books, which you may be interested about

Paleo Diet >>>>CLICK HERE<<<<

Air Fryer Recipes >>>>CLICK HERE<<<<

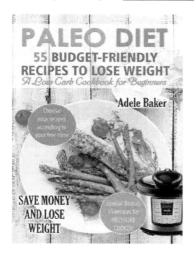 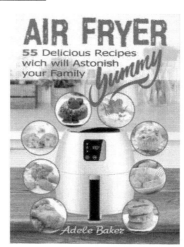

P.S. Thank you again for reading this book. If you've enjoyed it, please don't shy, drop me a line, leave a review or both on Amazon. I love reading your opinion; it helps me improve my book. Please share with me your success following this Keto diet.

Simply click HERE to leave the review!

Your Free Gift

Press the button below now and you will receive the next Cookbook of Pulsar Publishing Company for FREE.

http://bit.ly/2mfpWa9

I know you will love this gift!

Thanks and enjoy!

Made in the USA
Lexington, KY
27 August 2017